God's Pathway
to Healing

DIGESTION

BOOKS BY
REGINALD B. CHERRY, M.D.

―――――

GOD'S PATHWAY TO HEALING:

Digestion

Herbs That Heal

Joints and Arthritis

Menopause

Prostate

Vision

―――――

Dr. Cherry's Little Instruction Book

God's Pathway
to Healing

DIGESTION

by

Reginald B. Cherry, M.D.

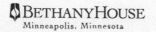
BETHANYHOUSE
Minneapolis, Minnesota

Published by Bethany House Publishers
A Ministry of Bethany Fellowship International
11400 Hampshire Avenue South
Bloomington, Minnesota 55438
www.bethanyhouse.com

Printed in the United States of America by
Bethany Press International,
Bloomington, Minnesota 55438

ISBN 0-7642-2766-1

CONTENTS

INTRODUCTION: TAKING CARE OF YOUR TEMPLE

Why are people with digestive problems swamping doctors' offices nationwide? In a recent year there were almost 38 million visits by patients with digestive disorders, and another 3.8 million went to hospital outpatient units, according to statistics published by the U.S. Department of Health and Human Services.

No doubt there were millions of other folks experiencing the same symptoms, pain, and discomfort, treating themselves with home remedies and over-the-counter medicines. Obviously, digestive tract ailments and diseases are a major American health concern.

Do *you* have good digestion?

How often do you have heartburn or indigestion? Do you suffer from gas, bloating, constipation, or diarrhea? Have you been diagnosed with ulcers, gastroesophageal reflux disease, or irritable bowel syndrome?

Are you tired all the time, with low energy? Have you killed off the "good bacteria" in your system, making you vulnerable to various infections—especially in these high-risk times when the whole world is worried about bioterrorism?

I'm not trying to alarm you unduly, but if you were concerned by any of the above questions, you need some authoritative medical answers and information. I have written this book to provide practical, commonsense advice that embraces up-to-date medical science, ancient spiritual truths from the Bible, and marvelous healing substances from natural sources.

There is help for you. I believe God wants you to be healthy and whole, and that you can find God's "pathway to healing"—a plan uniquely designed for your personal needs.

THE MASTER KEY TO HEALTH AND WELL-BEING

Of all the health essentials, digestion is perhaps the most basic. The truth is that

without a solid foundation of good digestion to provide proper nutrition for your
body, it is absolutely impossible to feel well
and be healthy.

The Bible declares in Proverbs 26:2
(KJV) that "the curse causeless shall not
come." I believe this simply means that
there is a reason why bad things happen.
In my years as a medical doctor, I've
learned that most digestive disorders can
be traced to poor eating habits and
improper nutrition. A diet of overly processed and refined foods that lack essential
nutrients such as fiber and enzymes can
result in a wide variety of intestinal disorders, including colon cancer.

Eating the proper foods in the right
amounts is so important that God listed in

the Bible what we should—and shouldn't—use for food. He sternly warned in Luke 21:34 (KJV): "Take heed to yourselves, lest at any time your hearts be overcharged with surfeiting [that's excessive overindulgence in something, like food], and drunkenness, and cares of this life [that's tension and stress]" (bracketed comments by author).

Americans are notorious for using the wrong foods, preparing them in the wrong way (with too much fat, rich sauces, and salt), and devouring far too much! Most restaurant portions are huge—two to three times more than a proper serving. Many fast-food chains even offer to "super-size" their burgers, fries, and soda for a few cents extra, so people consume more calories in one meal than their body typically needs all day!

Unquestionably, we live in a fast-paced, high-pressure world, trying to cram too much work and activity into each day. People stay on the go, "multitasking" (doing several things at once). Often they don't get enough rest . . . and eating on the run has become a way of life.

Along the journey, it's easy to forget the biblical warnings and fall deep into the very traps Jesus warned against. So here it is again—this time from the *Amplified Bible*: "Take heed to yourselves and be on your guard, lest your hearts be overburdened and depressed (weighed down) with the giddiness and headache and nausea of self-indulgence, drunkenness, and worldly worries and cares pertaining to (the business of) this life" (Luke 21:34).

MAKE TIME TO BE HEALTHY

However, it's not too late to make changes for the better. A good place to start may be to take a look at all you're doing now and begin to prioritize your activities. Maybe you think they are all good and worthwhile, but does that mean you have to do all of them at the same time?

Why not choose the best from the good, and make some time for *you*? It's hard to really enjoy life if it's rushing by so quickly that everything becomes a blur.

With some of the time you free up,

learn more about the marvelous temple God has given you to live in—your body. For example, the complex way our body processes food for nourishment and strength is truly remarkable. I want to stress the importance of what I call the *four primary principles of good digestion* that are vital to all of us. You can remember these four principles by using the simple acronym D-E-A-N. The D is for *digesting food,* the E is for *eliminating waste,* the A is for *absorbing nutrients,* and the N is for *normalizing the bacteria* in your colon.

This fourth principle is especially timely in this age of terrorism, with the renewed awareness of the threats of anthrax, tularemia, and other infectious agents that an enemy could use to try to wipe out entire cities. But did you know that the "good bacteria" in our digestive system provide a natural protective barrier between the outside world and the inner cellular working of our body? These "probiotic flora" are part of our frontline defense against invasive germ warfare.

In addition to helping you understand the miraculous workings of your digestive system, I also want to introduce you to the abundance of natural substances that can help you overcome any intestinal or digestive problems that may concern you now. Whether you suffer from indigestion and heartburn or a more threatening digestive disease, there is help and healing for you. We will look at the natural healers that are available in supplement form.

I'm glad you're joining me in this book in order to focus on some foundational truths about your health and, hopefully, to explore some new information that will lead you further along the road to divine abundance. Remember, God has a pathway to healing just for you, and He wants you to be well!

—Reginald B. Cherry, M.D.

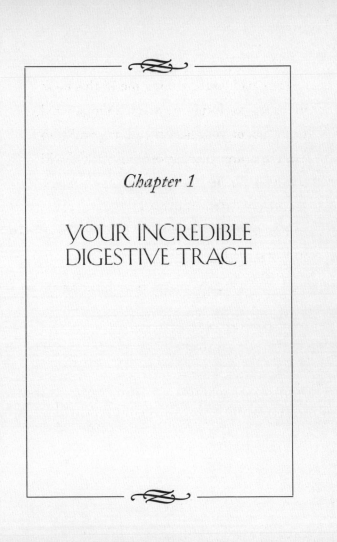

Chapter 1

YOUR INCREDIBLE
DIGESTIVE TRACT

Chapter 1

YOUR INCREDIBLE DIGESTIVE TRACT

It's a tube about thirty feet long that is tucked inside you, and when it doesn't function properly, you can get into big problems. We're talking about the digestive tract, which doctors generally call the gastrointestinal, or GI, tract. This tube digests food, absorbs water, secretes important enzymes, and essentially keeps us alive—and our body healthy.

The GI tract starts at the mouth and ends at the anal opening (I know you may not like to talk about this—but, hey, that's the way God made us). A constant, coordinated pattern of muscular contractions known as *peristalsis* moves food down the gastrointestinal tract. This wavelike motion is controlled by our automatic, or autonomic, involuntary nervous system. Normally it takes food from as little as twenty hours to as long as three or four days to pass through this muscular tube.

Digestion actually begins in the mouth as we chew, with our teeth mechanically breaking down food into small particles. An enzyme, amylase, is secreted in the saliva and mixed with the food to start breaking it down chemically.

Food quickly passes into the throat (or pharynx area) in just a few seconds, and then on into the esophagus. This tube is some ten inches long. Liquids pass right through it in only a few seconds, and the food mixture passes in about thirty seconds, and no more than a minute.

FIRST STOP—THE STOMACH

The food then progresses on to the stomach, first going through a small one-way valve designed to allow food to pass through but to stop the stomach's digestive acids from backing up into the esophagus. The wall of the stomach is protected from the acid by a lining of mucous, and the cells lining the stomach are actually replaced about every three days.

The esophagus has no such protection, so if the digestive acid does back up through a malfunctioning protective valve—a process called gastroesophageal reflux—the individual experiences the searing pain of heartburn or other potentially serious problems. Eating late at night and excessive weight gain are two major causes of valve failure and the resulting irritation and damage to the lower esophagus.

As the food arrives in the stomach, it is mixed with gastric juices and hydrochloric acid, which are designed to destroy bacteria and other potentially harmful organisms that might still be present. The food usually stays in the stomach about four hours, but it can remain for up to six or seven hours if it is made up of large amounts of fat, the most difficult substance to break down. This is why eating a large fatty meal late at night causes food to sit in your stomach for hours and can create a lot of misery.

Food exits the stomach through the pyloric valve. In some people, this valve does not open and close properly and prevents the stomach from emptying completely.

ENZYMES AND ENERGY

The pyloric valve opens into the first section of the small intestine, known as the duodenum. Food stays there about four hours while pancreatic enzymes are added to the mix to digest certain foods, and bile is added to further process fats. Later these secretions will help the rest of the small intestine and the large intestine to absorb the nutrients from the food.

As a person gets older, the pancreas may not produce as many of these enzymes as the body needs, which leads to incomplete digestion, a lack of energy, and possibly other ailments related to improper nourishment. This is why we recommend the use of a daily nutritional supplement containing certain enzymes.

After about four hours, the food passes farther into the small intestine to the jejunum area . . . then to the ileum, where the nutrients are absorbed through the walls of the tube into the bloodstream. This function may take another couple of hours or so.

The remaining food then passes into the colon, or large intestine. By this time most of the nutrients have been absorbed, except sodium and other salts, which are taken into the body through the colon. The nonabsorbed remainder is formed into a waste, or stool material. Water is taken out of this residue and absorbed, leaving a semisolid mass that will be moved to the rectum, a storage area for solid waste. This process takes about fourteen hours. The fecal matter ultimately will be gently expelled from the body through the anus in a bowel movement.

WHY YOU MAY NEED SUPPLEMENTS

Some of the most common problems patients consult their doctors about center around the GI tract, which certainly is understandable, given the complexity of this incredible system that is essential to our health and well-being. By attacking the GI tract, the enemy can keep food and nutrients from being absorbed and literally starve us to death, deprive us of energy, or cause numerous other maladies. Colon cancer, one of the most common cancers for both men and women, damages and destroys this vital organ of our body.

Other common diseases—diverticulosis and diverticulitis—involve inflammation of pouches in the lower colon. These disorders are related to insufficient fiber intake.

God has created a wonderful system that usually functions flawlessly. We can, however, do certain things to help our GI tract continue to work properly. For example, as we get older and begin to lose some of the digestive enzymes, we can use supplements that add enzymes like amylase, protease, lipase, cellulase, and others. Supplementing with substances such as cinnamon bark, fennel seed, and peppermint leaf powder is also helpful in maintaining our digestion and proper absorption of nutrients.

We all face potential attacks against our GI tract as we get older. Nevertheless, through supplements, timing our meals properly (that is, not eating late in the evening), and eating sufficient quantities of soluble and insoluble fiber, we can protect ourselves from most of the problems in the thirty-foot-long tube that is essential to our health.

Before we take a closer and more detailed look in the following chapters at what I call the four primary principles of good digestion, I'd like to lead you in a prayer for your digestive system. Rather than being a general "blanket" prayer, notice that this petition specifically addresses the various parts of your GI tract and focuses on each function, invoking supernatural assistance as well as divine direction to lead you into the personal pathway to healing God has for you. I recommend that you pray this prayer often in the days and weeks ahead as you move toward wholeness and perfect health.

MY PRAYER FOR THE GI TRACT

Father, I come to you in the name of Jesus, thanking you for the fearful and wonderful design of my body. I thank you for a healthy digestive system that will properly absorb the nutrients you created to bring strength, energy, and health to my body.

I pray specifically for healthy teeth, gums, and bone structure in my mouth to begin the digestion of my food. I thank you that my esophagus will contract normally, and I thank you that the valve at the end of my esophagus will close properly to prevent the backup of stomach acid, which can cause heartburn and scarring of tender tissue.

I thank you that my stomach will secrete proper amounts of acid and enzymes and that it will be free of bacteria that might cause peptic ulcer disease. Thank you that the valve that empties my stomach will function properly, preventing food from backing up in my stomach area.

Lord, I thank you for a healthy gallbladder that secretes bile and for a healthy pancreas that secretes the proper amounts of enzymes into my small intestine to digest and absorb the food that passes into it to provide nutrients and energy for my body.

I thank you for a healthy colon with cells that will remain free of abnormalities that could cause polyps or cancer. Thank you for *keeping my colon free of pockets that might become inflamed and that I will remain free of diverticulitis.*

I am so grateful that you have provided natural supplemental enzymes, and I pray that you will give me wisdom about consuming these, along with proper amounts of fiber, in addition to proper foods eaten at proper times to protect my digestive tract.

In Jesus' name, I declare myself free of digestive problems and diseases. As I do all that I know and am able to do in the natural, I will trust you, Father, to do all that I cannot do. In Jesus' name I pray all these things, in faith believing. Amen.

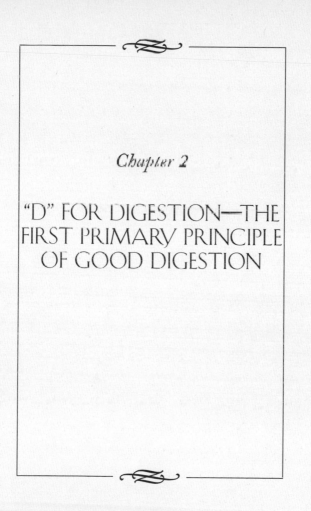

Chapter 2

"D" FOR DIGESTION—THE FIRST PRIMARY PRINCIPLE OF GOOD DIGESTION

Chapter 2

"D" FOR DIGESTION—THE FIRST PRIMARY PRINCIPLE OF GOOD DIGESTION

Perhaps more than any other profession, the practice of medicine requires never-ending, ongoing study and research. Not only do we live in an age of rapidly changing technology and pharmaceuticals, with new diagnostic equipment and drugs becoming available every year, but medical research teams are constantly questioning, re-verifying, and refining virtually all basic medical knowledge.

In addition, they are conducting exhaustive tests of hundreds of vitamins, herbs, minerals, foods, and various natural substances that are now available for use as supplements or alternative treatment options. Some of these have been known and used as folk remedies for centuries but were largely ignored by most medical practitioners. Now it seems that increasing numbers within the medical community are paying serious new attention to these substances, and they are even beginning to combine them with more conventional treatment options.

I spend many hours every week reading medical journals and studying test results that are being reported by research scientists on university and independent Internet sites. Sometimes the sheer volume of new information is almost overwhelming. Often the new studies confirm truths that God recorded in His Word thousands of years ago.

WALKING IN THE FOOTSTEPS OF GOD

A great deal of the information we are discovering in science today parallels and bolsters what the Bible says about nutrition, hygiene, and basic health practices. In fact, science is walking in the footsteps of God, still catching up with His grand design and reconfirming the ancient laws the Lord gave His people thirty-five centuries ago.

The Living Bible declares in Proverbs 24:3: "Any enterprise is built by wise planning, becomes strong through common sense, and profits wonderfully by keeping abreast of the facts." This certainly is true in today's world of medicine.

As I said earlier, digestive problems rank as one of the major reasons people go to doctors' offices today. In addition to disorders such as indigestion, heartburn, bloating, gas, constipation, and diarrhea, the GI tract can develop even more serious problems, such as peptic ulcers, reflux disease, irritable bowel syndrome, and even colon cancer.

Largely because of the increased research being done, medical science has come a long way in only the last couple of years toward a better understanding of digestion. We have a much better idea of how our body is supposed to work, why things go wrong, and what can be done to correct the problems and avoid their re-occurrence.

This brings us to the new emphasis on what I call the four primary principles of good digestion. Essentially, this involves *digesting*, or breaking down, the food we eat, *eliminating* the waste products that accumulate, *absorbing* the nutrients from the food, and *normalizing* the balance of good bacteria, or flora, that God created to reside naturally inside the colon. It's important to understand these four principles, and again, a simple tool to help remember them is the use of the acronym D-E-A-N.

THE KEYS TO GOOD DIGESTION

In this chapter we are dealing with D, for digestion. We've already seen that chewing our food mechanically breaks it into smaller pieces, and that the acid and bile in the stomach further break down the food chemically to a semiliquid state. Even so, the real work of digestion, getting the food into a form that can be absorbed by the body, takes place in the small intestine.

The food mixture that floods into the small intestine from the stomach is known as *chyme*. As it begins passing through the duodenum, most of the water and electrolytes—including sodium, chloride, and potassium—are absorbed through the wall of the small intestine into the bloodstream. Also, most of the dietary organic molecules are further digested, including glucose, amino acids, and fatty acids.

The digestive process in the small intestine not only provides essential nutrients to the body but also plays a critical role in water and acid-base balance, which is vital to good health.

The key ingredients that accomplish this are enzymes secreted by the pancreas. Among the key enzymes are:

Amylase, which chews up carbohydrates, converting them from the more complex plant starch forms into more simple saccharides, or sugar forms.

Proteolytic enzymes, or *proteases,* break down protein, one of the hardest substances for the body to digest. An enzyme called *trypsin* also helps break down complex proteins into simple amino acids through a process known as hydrolysis, which uses water molecules to break the bond that holds amino acids together.

Lipase is the enzyme that dissolves fats. The major form of dietary fat is triglyceride, and before it can be directly absorbed through the mucous wall of the intestine, it must be separated into its component parts, a monoglyceride and two free fatty acids. Sufficient quantities of bile salts from the liver must also be present to break down triglycerides and prepare the fatty acids and monoglycerides to be absorbed by the body to use as fuel and energy.

Incidentally, pancreatic lipase has been the focus of recent studies as a possible tool in the management of obesity. A drug called *Orlistat* is a pancreatic lipase inhibitor that interferes with the digestion of triglyceride and reduces the absorption of dietary fat. Researchers believe that inhibiting lipase may lead to significant reductions in body weight in some patients.

These three primary enzyme groups—amylase, proteases, and lipase—enable the body to digest the four major food groups: grains and breads, fruits and vegetables, milk and dairy, and meat and fish.

THE CRUCIAL ROLE OF THE PANCREAS

While various enzymes are produced in different areas of the digestive tract, they primarily occur in the first half of the small intestine. As mentioned, these enzymes are secreted by the pancreas—a long, pinkish-white organ about the size of a small banana that sits below the liver and behind the stomach. In addition to the digestive breakdown of proteins, fats, and starch into a form that can be absorbed, the pancreas has another crucial role. Its first order of business at this stage of the digestive process is to quickly and efficiently neutralize the stomach acid in the chyme to keep it from attacking and damaging the small intestine.

Then comes the secretion of enzymes to change the molecular nutrients into a form that can be absorbed into the blood. Every day the pancreas secretes about a quart and a half of pancreatic juice, containing about fifteen enzymes, into the small intestine. Without this function of the pancreas, our bodies would literally starve to death, even if they were consuming adequate quantities of high-quality food. Imagine the energy load and stress on the pancreas to produce and secrete enough of the various enzymes required to process the volume and different types of food the body takes in each day.

These digestive enzymes are absolutely critical. If the pancreas slows down or produces a limited amount of enzymes, digestion is affected and hampered. What are the symptoms? Immediate discomfort, with possible bloating, gas buildup, constipation, or diarrhea, because the food passes through the GI tract only partially digested, or not at all.

For example, if an insufficient amount of the enzyme *lactase* is supplied, the body cannot tolerate milk and dairy products, which normally are broken down into a carbohydrate called lactose. About 20 percent of the population is milk-intolerant and must avoid the important dairy foods.

Another enzyme that deals with carbohydrates is *cellulase,* which breaks down the cell walls of various plants and vegetables ordinarily used for food. With too little cellulase, the cell walls remain intact and there can be no digestion. The resulting waste mass must be expelled from the digestive system, which can be a thoroughly unpleasant experience for the body's owner.

If the pancreas produces an insufficient amount of *proteolytic* enzymes, protein digestion is affected. As we have seen, proteins are one of the more difficult substances for the body to digest, and without enough enzymes, these essential nutrients are lost. Even worse than losing the nourishment, undigested proteins may even do damage to the body.

One theory, called the "leaky gut syndrome," suggests that if large protein molecules are not broken down properly into amino acids by the proteases, they migrate farther into the gut and pass through the wall of the intestine into the bloodstream. Proponents of this still-unproven theory feel that protein migration may prompt the body to create antibodies that can cause allergies and maybe even contribute to arthritis in some cases.

"WHY DON'T I HAVE MORE ENERGY?"

Whether or not the leaky gut syndrome proves to be valid, another major problem definitely occurs when the pancreas does not produce enough enzymes for efficient, complete digestion: the body does not get the energy it needs to function properly. Without the fuel to sustain an adequate energy level, extreme fatigue starts shutting down the body. With constant fatigue, the body becomes more vulnerable to dysfunction and disease and less able to defend and heal itself.

The pancreas performs another critically important function for the welfare of the body. In addition to being an *exocrine* organ—producing a secretion that goes outside itself to an exterior organ—the pancreas is also an *endocrine* organ that secretes major hormones internally through the bloodstream. The pancreas provides insulin and glucagons, which are essential to the body's metabolism (or use) of carbohydrates and fats. Insulin and glucagons are necessary for maintaining normal blood-sugar levels.

There is something we can do to help boost the enzyme level in our digestive tract, improving the body's digestion and enhancing the metabolic processes. We can assist the pancreas by eating a well-balanced diet of nutritionally sound foods, and by increasing our body's supply of the crucial digestive enzymes in supplement form.

As we know, enzymes play an important role in facilitating the body's vital metabolic processes: digesting foods, purifying the blood, providing energy, and getting rid of waste. There are multiple sources of these enzymes in addition to those produced by the body.

Many uncooked plant foods contain enzymes that can aid digestion. These food-borne enzymes ease the need for digestive enzymes by predigesting foods as they sit in the stomach. By the time foods reach the small intestine, fewer internally produced enzymes are needed to finish the digestive process.[1]

For example, papaya and pineapple are two of the richest plant sources of proteolytic enzymes, which help digest the proteins in food. You may be aware that they have traditionally been used as natural tenderizers for meat. *Papain* and *bromelain* are the respective names for the enzymes found in these fruits.

Many practitioners of alternative medicine believe that proteolytic enzymes can be helpful for a wide variety of other health conditions, including food allergies and autoimmune diseases. Scientific studies and tests have shown that controlled use of these enzymes improves the rate of healing of sports injuries, promotes faster recovery from surgery, and aids in treating bruises as well as the painful condition known as shingles (*herpes zoster*).

Enzymes cannot only be added through the diet, they can also be taken as a supplement in capsule form, usually taken just before eating. Orally ingested enzymes can bypass the conditions of the GI tract and be absorbed into the bloodstream while still maintaining their enzymatic activity. In addition to proteolytic enzymes, lipases, and amylases, ginger is often recommended. Ginger has been used throughout history as an aid for many gastrointestinal disturbances and as a tonic for the digestive tract.

FEARFULLY AND WONDERFULLY MADE

Did you have any idea how unbelievably complex and amazing your digestive system is? We are walking miracles, all of us! No wonder the psalmist exclaimed, "I praise you because I am fearfully and wonderfully made" (139:14 NIV).

In the next chapter, we will look into another of the four primary principles of good digestion: *elimination*—how your body handles waste. I think you will be impressed—maybe even amazed—at how important this function is to your body's health and to your general well-being.

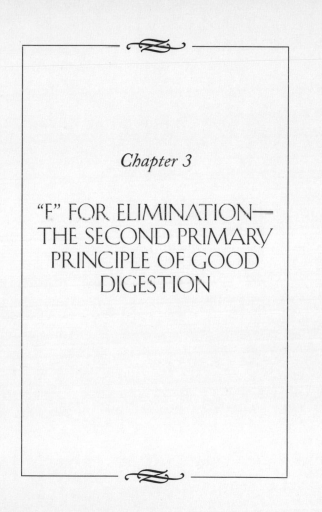

Chapter 3

"F" FOR ELIMINATION— THE SECOND PRIMARY PRINCIPLE OF GOOD DIGESTION

Chapter 3

"E" FOR ELIMINATION—THE SECOND PRIMARY PRINCIPLE OF GOOD DIGESTION

Once the first step in the digestive process is complete—the breaking down of food nutrients into a simple sugar form that can be absorbed and used by the body—the gastrointestinal tract immediately and efficiently goes to work eliminating the remaining waste products.

We've already seen how the GI tract

extracts protein, vitamins, minerals, and other nutrients from the food, leaving the waste material in the bowels. The colon absorbs much of the remaining salts and leftover water, and then pushes the waste farther down toward the rectum by a process of muscular contractions called peristaltic waves.

The waste is formed into a semisolid mass, or stool material. Ultimately the fecal matter will be expelled in a bowel movement. Regular bowel action is very important to move the waste out of the body as soon as possible. The less time the stool stays in the colon the better, so that fewer toxins, or poisons, can attack the GI tract.

Again, on the average, the process of

removing the excess water from the waste and moving it to the rectum takes about fourteen hours. Bowel movements differ according to each person and do not necessarily occur daily. The "norm" may range from twice a day to three or four times a week.

STOPPING UP THE WORKS

If the rate of waste moving through the colon slows down, an excess amount of water may be extracted, leaving the fecal material dry and hard. This is known as constipation, which can be very uncomfortable. Often the person feels bloated or "gassy," and bowel movements are painful, with cramping and straining that can lead to the development of hemorrhoids.

Normal regularity can be slowed by a wide range of causes, including stress, illness, travel, pregnancy, sitting for long periods of time, an overall lack of adequate exercise, not drinking enough water, and certain medications. Far and away the most common cause, though, is a lack of fiber in the diet.

If elimination slows down until it actually stops, there can be the potentially dangerous condition of an impacted colon. This can be very serious because it shuts down the complex functioning of the GI tract, especially the providing of fuel and energy to the body. Obviously, this condition requires immediate medical attention.

Many people who experience frequent

constipation resort to the use of drugstore over-the-counter laxatives. I don't recommend this practice because some laxatives are harsh enough to damage the lining of the GI tract and, at best, may cause an individual to become dependent on this aid. The healthiest laxative for occasional use is a magnesium-based product like Milk of Magnesia.

Certain foods, such as prunes, raisins, and figs, are natural laxatives that increase the moisture content of the stool and make passage easier. Drinking plenty of liquids daily—water, fruit, and vegetable juices— also aids in elimination. A word of caution: these fruits and most fruit juices are also high in calories and can elevate blood-sugar levels.

Personally, I eat a high-fiber cereal almost daily, which helps with regularity and also helps keep my cholesterol level low. Kellogg's Bran Buds is a mixture of different types of fiber—water-soluble psyllium plus water-insoluble wheat bran. This cereal is crunchy and tastes good. Another one I recommend is a mixture of a half cup of Fiber One cereal with a third cup of oat bran. Use skim or one-half-percent low-fat milk, or substitute soymilk.

For a snack, try psyllium wafers (my favorite is cinnamon spice). They contain significant amounts of psyllium but taste good. Be sure to drink a full glass of water with them.

Another natural and effective treatment for constipation is getting a reasonable amount of exercise every day, such as taking a brisk twenty minute walk. Equally important is selecting a healthy diet, avoiding highly processed junk foods, and consuming adequate amounts of fiber. We'll talk about this in more detail later.

THE MISERY OF IBS

Irritable bowel syndrome, or IBS (formerly known as spastic colon), is an extremely common problem. In fact, it is the number one referral by family physicians to gastroenterologists and affects millions of people.

Symptoms include abdominal bloating and cramping, gas, and either diarrhea or constipation, or alternating between the two. The exact physical cause still has not been identified, but it appears to be a problem with the transmission of nerve impulses to the smooth muscles in the GI tract. Stress is a significant factor contributing to this condition.

In severe cases of IBS, medications that relax the smooth muscles in the GI tract may be effective for relieving abdominal pain and discomfort. However, excellent results are also being obtained with the use of peppermint oil (available in capsule form), which tends to stop the excessive spasms in the colon's smooth muscle.

The British medical journal *Lancet* described a controlled test that reported a nearly 50 percent reduction in colon spasms in patients who used one or two

0.2-milligram peppermint oil capsules a day. *Caution:* Peppermint oil must be taken in capsule form, as it can relax the sphincter muscle between the stomach and the esophagus and cause acid reflux.

Other effective treatments for irritable bowel syndrome include psyllium and wheat bran—remember, both are found in the breakfast cereal Bran Buds (try about a quarter cup with low-fat milk).

HAVE YOU HAD YOUR FIBER TODAY?

The key to helping your intestines and colon stay healthy is to eat more fiber! God put this essential component into the basic and best foods He provided for people at the dawn of creation in the Garden of

Eden (see Genesis 1:11–12). This means our diet should include plenty of vegetables and fruits and a reasonable amount of grains. Eating the right kinds of foods in the proper quantities provides the vitamins and nutrients necessary for health and strength and also promotes healthy, normal elimination.

The bottom line is that it really does matter what you eat. It also matters how you eat it. Vegetables should be eaten raw, if possible, or at least cooked only slightly, since cooking may soften and degrade the fiber. Don't peel fruits like apples and pears, because much of the fiber is in the skin. Beans and other legumes, which are high in fiber content, should be added to soups, stews, and salads.

Most Americans are fiber deficient. Eating white flour, white rice, fruit juice instead of fruit, and other highly processed foods all contribute to the problem. The typical modern Western diet provides approximately ten grams of fiber per day. So-called primitive societies consume forty to sixty grams per day.[1]

Several years ago a study was done that compared the diet and elimination of rural African tribesmen with a group of British naval officers. The Africans' natural diet provided more than one hundred grams of fiber per day and, not surprisingly, they had regular bowel movements and virtually no digestive complaints or food-related conditions or diseases.

The naval officers ate mainly meats,

sugar, and white flour and complained of poor digestion and frequent constipation. The British also developed hemorrhoids, diverticulitis and diverticulosis, hiatal hernias, high cholesterol, irritable bowel syndrome, high blood pressure, diabetes, and colon and rectal cancer.[2]

Fiber is divided into two general categories—water-soluble and water-insoluble. Soluble fibers lower blood cholesterol and delay glucose absorption, which lowers blood-sugar levels in people with diabetes. Insoluble fiber speeds the transit time of food passing through the GI tract, softening the stool and increasing the fecal weight, both important benefits for better waste elimination. Both types of fiber help fill the stomach, reducing appetite. In theory, this should reduce eating and lead to weight loss.

Whole grains are particularly high in insoluble fiber. Oats, barley, beans, fruit (but not fruit juice), psyllium, and some vegetables contain significant amounts of both forms of fiber and are the best sources of soluble fiber.

Fiber has been shown to provide significant treatment benefits for constipation, diabetes, diverticular diseases, high cholesterol, and obesity, and is also believed to help with diarrhea, hemorrhoids, and high blood pressure. It is also beneficial for conditions such as high triglycerides, irritable bowel syndrome, kidney stones, peptic ulcers, and premenstrual syndrome.

GLUCOMANNAN!

In the last couple of years there has been a tremendous influx of research information about the digestive tract, probably because digestive disorders have become a primary medical problem. I have spent a great deal of time reviewing various tests, studies, and reports in medical journals.

During my research, I became intrigued with a unique fiber from Japan called *glucomannan*. For many years the Japanese have made a flour from the konjac root and also a jelly called konyaku, which is a common and popular food product.

Perhaps it is just a coincidence that the residents of certain Japanese island groups have the longest life span of any group of people in the world. Even so, the unique health benefits of this water-soluble fiber—glucomannan—certainly couldn't hurt their longevity.

Glucomannan is in the same class of fibers as pectin, a fiber gel commonly used in making jellies and jams. Its uniqueness comes from the fact that it can absorb *seventeen times* its volume of water—that's *two hundred times* its weight in water! This is very significant.

All water-soluble fibers absorb water, but none of them to that extent. This means that when used as an aid to the digestive system, a much smaller quantity of glucomannan could be used than, say, psyllium or oat bran.

Commercial formulas of water-soluble fibers require mixing a packet of powder in a big glass of water, stirring it up, and *yuk*! The stuff doesn't taste so hot! A tiny amount of glucomannan can be put into a capsule and swallowed. Inside the stomach, the powder mixes with the water already there and quickly forms a gelatinous mass.

Even a small quantity of this substance can turn into an absolute powerhouse in absorbing water, balancing cholesterol, and creating a feeling of fullness in the stomach. Research is now being done using glucomannan as part of a weight-loss supplement, since it has no calories and provides volume and fullness that could help suppress appetite. The fiber also slows down the body's absorption of sugar, which tends to regulate the spiking, or wide fluctuations, in blood-sugar levels. Obviously, this can be a great benefit to diabetics.

Glucomannan not only lowers the total cholesterol count, but it also promotes balance by raising the HDL, or good, cholesterol while lowering the LDL, or bad, cholesterol. It also brings better balance to the nutrients going into the bloodstream by the absorption of bile acids and salts in the colon.

The gel-like mass formed in the stomach moves on into the GI tract and is ultimately compacted and mixed with the stool. Its high water volume allows it to function as a stool softener, an excellent quality for people who suffer from constipation and hard stools.

Any substance that helps overcome irregularity in elimination can be a valuable aid to colon health. Limiting the transit time of food passing through the colon and shortening the length of time the stool remains there obviously cuts down on the amount of exposure the colon wall has to the toxins that occur in the stool.[3]

I'm excited about the increased knowledge and new breakthroughs in the area of colon health. With the ability to supplement the body's access to digestive enzymes, to restore and balance the good bacteria (or flora, which we'll talk about in detail in chapter five), and to put special types of super-absorbent fiber into supplement form, there is something we can do to enjoy better digestion. There's really no reason why any of us has to suffer from digestive problems any longer.

The apostle John wrote, "Beloved, I pray that you may prosper in every way and (that your body) may keep well, even as (I know) your soul keeps well and prospers" (3 John 2 AMP).

Truly, God is showing us the way to health and well-being in these last days.

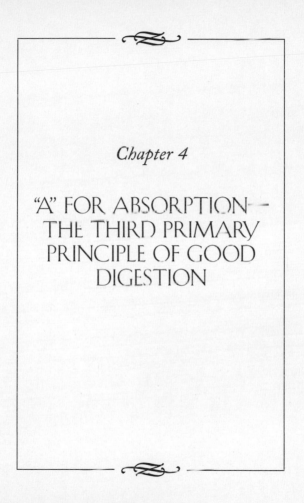

Chapter 4

"A" FOR ABSORPTION – THE THIRD PRIMARY PRINCIPLE OF GOOD DIGESTION

Chapter 4

"A" FOR ABSORPTION—THE THIRD PRIMARY PRINCIPLE OF GOOD DIGESTION

Perhaps you've heard people say, "You are what you eat." That may be a catchy phrase, but it isn't entirely true. A more accurate, though less memorable, statement might be "You are what your body digests and absorbs."

Even if we plan our diets and eat the proper foods our body needs, our efforts won't do any good *unless* the food is digested *and* absorbed into the bloodstream. Only then can the nutrients be distributed to the cells that make up various organs and used for fuel to operate the complex systems of the body.

I've had patients tell me, "What I eat doesn't seem to do me any good"—and they were right. Although they were eating enough to fuel the body, the food was not being properly digested, with little or incomplete absorption of nutrients. As a result, their bodies were in starvation mode, causing them to feel draggy and tired all the time, with low energy.

As we have been saying, the four primary principles of good digestion can be remembered by using the acronym

D-E-A-N. Digestion, Elimination, Absorption, and Normalizing the bacteria in the colon are all essential to good nutrition and good health.

God has designed our body to efficiently process the food we take in by breaking it down into smaller, simpler molecules that provide nourishment to be converted into energy to give us strength and keep us going. This really is nothing short of miraculous, considering the fact that most of the food we eat would be as deadly as poison if it went directly into our bloodstream.

YOUR GUT FEEDS YOU

You've probably heard people use the slang expression "feeding my gut" in reference to eating. Actually it's the other way around: your gut feeds you. The whole GI tract can be described as an elaborate food "disassembly" plant.

Except for dietary fibers like bran, nut husks, celery strings, etc., your gut disassembles virtually everything you eat into smaller components the body needs and can use. It converts the protein from your roast beef dinner into smaller amino acids that can be used to build and repair body tissues. It changes the large carbohydrates in your mashed potatoes into sugary glucose, which is a rich source of energy for the body. The process of using powerful tools called enzymes to break down complex food elements into simpler nutrients is called digestion.

Without the miracle of the digestive process, you would soon starve to death no matter how much you gorged yourself. So your gut feeds you. Which brings us to *absorption,* the process by which the products of digestion are transferred into the body's internal environment, enabling them to reach the cells.

THE BODY'S "HAPPENING PLACE"

Nutrient absorption takes place in the middle of the abdomen, in the twenty-foot-long small intestine. Divided into three sections—the duodenum, jejunum, and ileum—the mid-gut absorbs the nutrients, vitamins, and minerals from the up to two gallons of food, liquid, and digestive secretions the body takes in every day.

The duodenum, a section about two feet long between the stomach and the jejunum, is a very active place. Through muscular contractions that create a to-and-fro motion, the food and enzymes are further mixed to encourage continued, complete digestion.

The jejunum and its lining handle the task of absorption—the passing of digested molecules of food through cell membranes into the blood or lymph capillaries—where they are carried off in the bloodstream to other parts of the body. Every square inch of the intestinal wall is covered with tiny fingerlike protusions called *villi*, themselves covered with about ten billion microscopic hairlike projections called *microvilli,* which actually absorb nutrients into your bloodstream

Only God could have envisioned and designed such an unbelievably compact and complex organism. Consider this: if the inside of your gut were smooth, there would only be about six square feet of absorptive surface. Instead, with the folds, villi, and microvilli, there are about *four thousand* square feet—about the same surface as two tennis courts![1]

The jejunum specializes in the absorption of carbohydrates and proteins, which happens in the first foot or two of this segment of the intestine—usually about five feet in total length. The ileum, the bottom segment of the small intestine, handles the absorption of water, fats, and bile salts.

TAKE A MOMENT TO
CONSIDER THE LIVER

Where does the nutrient-rich blood go after it absorbs the digested food from the gut? To the liver, which receives blood flowing from the intestine toward the heart. The liver's function is to further process the material that has been absorbed from the intestinal tract so that the cells in the body can utilize it. For example, it produces sugars from proteins and fatty substances. Also, the liver is a storage organ for specialized materials such as Vitamin B12 (important in making red blood cells) and sugars that fuel the contraction of muscles and other cellular functions.

The liver also deals with toxic substances circulating in the bloodstream, converting them into materials that can safely be excreted from the body. It does all these things—and more—at an incredible speed.[2]

What's left over in the gut after all this processing and absorption is an indigestible watery waste that passes on into the colon (or large intestine). The main job here is to reclaim the excess water from the intestinal waste and recycle it back into the bloodstream for reuse. Someone has described the colon's function as a "water treatment plant." The remaining solid sludge, or stool, moves on to the rectum for final elimination as a bowel movement.

We noted earlier that without the normal function of the absorption process, the body would not receive proper nutrition, and it would go into starvation mode. Without enough fuel for energy, essential bodily functions in various organs would slow or shut down. In addition to feeling tired and lethargic, barely able to go on, the undernourished body also becomes susceptible both to organic malfunction and to attacks from bacteria, viruses, and other destructive forces as the immune system begins to weaken.

WHEN THINGS GO WRONG

The small intestine has two major functions. The first is to allow necessary substances into the bloodstream in order for the body to use these raw materials to grow and function properly. With the aid of enzymes (found in pancreatic juices and secretions from the small intestine), sugars, amino acids, fats, vitamins, minerals, and other food factors are processed into small molecules that can safely pass into the bloodstream. If this process fails, the patient is said to have a malabsorption syndrome.

The second major function of the small intestine is a protective one—preventing toxic substances and large molecules from getting into the bloodstream. These large molecules —such as protein molecules— cannot be handled well by the body and can cause the immune system to produce antibodies against them.[3]

If large molecules are absorbed through the intestine into the bloodstream, this increased intestinal permeability, or leaky gut syndrome, can cause all kinds of problems. Some medical researchers believe these may include immunological disorders such as inflammatory and infectious bowel diseases, some forms of chronic arthritis, and skin conditions like acne and psoriasis.

The leaky gut itself may be caused by food allergy reactions, infections, or toxic agents. While there are differing schools of thought about the causes and effects of intestinal permeability (or leaky gut syndrome), the problem is very real to its sufferers. Once this condition is identified, it is important to correct the cause or causes and also to attempt to repair the damage to the intestine.

SIMPLE THINGS YOU CAN DO TO HELP

If you're having digestive problems—especially if you suspect your nutrient absorption is not up to par—be sure to consult your doctor and share your symptoms and the way you feel. Don't be embarrassed to describe the difficulties you're experiencing. It won't be the first time he or she has heard about the problem, and knowing the details will be very beneficial to your doctor in helping you find your pathway to healing.

In addition to medical assistance, there are some simple, commonsense things you can do. The chances are very high that you could add more fiber to your diet . . . and drink more water. Most people don't get enough of either! And getting at least twenty minutes of basic exercise per day can do nothing but improve your health, even if you do as little as take a couple of brisk ten-minute walks each day.

Try limiting "trouble" foods in your diet: sugars, starches, fruit juices, and "gassy" foods such as milk and dairy products. If you're not sure what you're eating, try writing down every bite of food you put into your mouth for a few days. You might be surprised at how little or how much of certain foods you are consuming. Your doctor would also like to see that food diary.

Consider supplementing your regular food intake with some natural substances such as herbs, vitamins, and minerals. For example, garlic and oregano are both available in tablet form and have proven to be helpful to many people with poor digestion.

Also, hawthorn can be an important supplement for individuals concerned about absorption and assimilation of nutrients. If your digestion seems sluggish and your abdomen feels tight and distended, hawthorn can help by stimulating enzymes involved in fat and protein digestion—from foods like meat—and to curb the appetite.

Hawthorn has been used in China since ancient times for digestion, and Europeans since the Renaissance have used it for digestive ailments. As a bonus, hawthorn is also believed to treat heart disease by strengthening cardiac muscle contraction.

Finally, take time to pray. God made your body, and He can fix it! I recommend that you use the prayer at the end of chapter 1 because it is specific, but feel free to simply talk to God and tell Him exactly how you are feeling and what you would like Him to do. Ask for His help, His direction, and His guidance. He will hear you, and He will answer!

Be sure to listen for His voice.

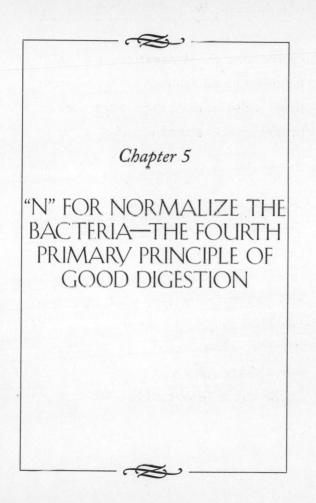

Chapter 5

"N" FOR NORMALIZE THE BACTERIA—THE FOURTH PRIMARY PRINCIPLE OF GOOD DIGESTION

Chapter 5

"N" FOR NORMALIZE THE BACTERIA—THE FOURTH PRIMARY PRINCIPLE OF GOOD DIGESTION

Perhaps there has never been a time in the history of the world when we've needed a hedge of protection around our body more than we do now. After the massive terrorist strikes that leveled the twin towers of New York's World Trade Center and damaged the Pentagon in Washington, D.C., Americans, especially, began to realize how vulnerable we are to attack.

The awful breakouts of the anthrax virus in various parts of the country, presumably distributed via the mail, vividly demonstrated that the long-dreaded use of bacterial and infective agents in terrorism and biological warfare is both possible and deadly. Sadly, we now can envision the population of entire cities being stricken by killer bacteria in the water supply, or the whole world being put in peril by the deliberate reintroduction of a once-conquered plague like smallpox.

No wonder Jesus warned that in the last days there would be "famines and pestilences (plagues, malignant and contagious or infectious epidemic diseases, deadly and devastating)" (Luke 21:11 AMP). Earlier in that chapter He said, "Be on your guard" (v. 8). I believe one way we can do that naturally is by fortifying our body, and we'll be talking about this further.

First, though, the Bible also has great words of encouragement for us: "Thou wilt keep him in perfect peace, whose mind is stayed on thee: because he trusteth in thee" (Isaiah 26:3 KJV).

"Be careful for nothing; but in every thing by prayer and supplication with thanksgiving let your requests be made known unto God. And the peace of God, which passeth all understanding, shall keep your hearts and minds through Christ Jesus" (Philippians 4:6–7 KJV).

WHAT DOES ALL THIS HAVE TO DO WITH DIGESTION?

Nothing ever sneaks up on the Lord! He says, "I am God, and there is none like Me, declaring the end from the beginning, and from ancient times things that are not yet done" (Isaiah 46:9–10 NKJV).

He made provision for the events of the last days at the dawn of creation when He formed man from the dust of the earth.

God designed the digestive tract to selectively absorb the things that are beneficial for us and to eliminate those things that are bad for us. The amazingly complex GI tract is a natural barrier between the outside world and the inner cellular workings of the body. Believe it or not, the front line of defense against unwelcome foreign invaders of the body are the good bacteria that dwell in the colon: more than four hundred species of "beneficial bugs" that oppose and attack bad bacteria while supporting and fostering healthy life in the very core of the body.

Get this: the good bacteria (or flora) in our gut are described as *probiotic*, which literally means "pro-life." Two of the main pro-life forces in the colon are known as *bifidobacterium bifidum* and *lactobacillus acidophilus*. They help balance the intestinal microflora by stopping or slowing the growth of harmful bacteria, promoting good digestion, boosting immune function, and increasing resistance to infection.

For example, acidophilus and bifidobacteria produce organic compounds such as lactic acid, hydrogen peroxide, and acetic acid, which increase the acid level of the intestine enough to slow the reproduction of many harmful bacteria. In fact, medical researchers believe that enhancing the acidic environment of the colon protects against and decreases the risk of colon cancer.

Probiotic bacteria also produce other substances that act as natural antibiotics to kill undesirable microorganisms. As a result, they have been shown to be effective in preventing vaginal infections, especially yeast infections. There is always a certain amount of yeast in the body, but with the proper amount of good bacteria present, yeast colonization does not occur.[1]

HOW "PRO-LIFE" BACTERIA PROTECT YOU

Did you know that the majority of our immune system is actually located in the lining of our small intestine? It's true, and with the right balance of probiotics versus bad bacteria in the GI tract, the immune system is strengthened. If ever there was a time when we needed to strengthen our immune system, it's now, with the ominous threat of bioterrorism attack. Our bodies need to be at their peak of resistance to help protect us from anthrax, tularemia, and various other onslaughts of bacterial infections that might occur.

At the same time, with the good bacteria in our colon actually producing natural antibiotic substances, our bodies are better equipped to deal with various other health challenges. Probiotics may be helpful for preventing different types of diarrhea—infectious or "travel" diarrhea, antibiotic-induced diarrhea, and childhood diarrhea. They may also generally improve the health of the gastrointestinal system. Acidophilus, for example, is a source of lactase, the enzyme needed to digest milk, which is lacking in many people.

Probiotic treatment has also been proposed for canker sores, Crohn's disease, eczema symptoms in infants, and as a treatment for people with irritable bowel syndrome.

In short, probiotics are good for you. The more good bacteria you have in your colon, the more resistant you are to infection and the more you can overcome bad bacteria that might invade your body.

BE CAREFUL WITH ANTIBIOTICS!

Just as probiotic means "pro-life," the word antibiotic technically means "against life," or "anti-life." Occasionally a person may have a legitimate need to take a pre-scribed antibiotic medicine to treat pneu-monia or a sinus or bronchial infection. The antibiotic effectively kills bad bacteria, which cause the infection or disease; it works.

But while it is killing the bad bacteria, the antibiotic wipes out good "pro-life" bac-teria in the colon as well, leaving the gut vul-nerable and unprotected. When this happens, other harmful bacteria and yeast can soon move back in and flourish. That's why some people get a yeast infection following a round of antibiotics.

To make matters worse, a growing number of patients want their doctor to prescribe an antibiotic for them at the first sign of sickness, even conditions their body might well be able to handle without medication. Some healthy people even ask for prescriptions for antibiotics just to have on hand in case they get sick! Some even take them when they don't have an infection, which does them far more harm than good.

In addition to killing off the probiotic flora, overuse of antibiotics seems to promote the emergence of "super bacteria," which develop an immunity to antibiotics.

Drug companies have formulated different types of antibiotics in stronger, more powerful dosages to try to combat these new strains of bacteria.

You might think, *Well, that doesn't apply to me, because I haven't been on antibiotics for anything lately.* Interestingly enough, most of us are getting an antibiotic buildup whether we take prescription drugs or not. We get it from poultry, dairy products, and meat, because farmers now regularly use antibiotics in animal feed to protect their flocks and herds from infectious microbes.

People take in trace amounts of antibiotics almost daily, even when they try to eat healthy. They can't see them. They can't smell them. They can't taste them. Yet every bite they take is killing off the good bacteria in their colon that they vitally need.

Then, for the last fifteen years or so, a growing number of practitioners have promoted the use of colon washes (or hydrotherapy), colon irrigation, high enemas, and the like. In addition to washing away good and bad bacteria alike—leaving the colon defenseless from invasive attack—there is a risk that the mechanics of these washing practices can damage the soft tissue of the anus and lower colon.

HAVE YOU HAD YOUR YOGURT TODAY?

Any time a person has been put on an antibiotic for any reason, the colon needs to be repopulated with good bacteria to replace those that were destroyed by the medication. I can't overemphasize the necessity of normalizing the flora in the colon. Simply add live probiotic bacteria cultures that will reproduce and bring back balance to the colon.

There are various supplements available that are supposed to have live cultures of good bacteria. Nevertheless, one of the easiest, most convenient, and most economical ways to get the job done is to eat yogurt, a folk remedy used for hundreds, if not thousands, of years. I'm not talking about the frozen dessert kind, but the natural sour custard that has live cultures of bacteria in it.

This is so important, that I recommend adding a serving of a good quality yogurt to your daily diet to keep the proper balance of

good bacteria in your system. Because probiotics are not drugs but are living organisms
you're trying to transplant into your digestive
tract, it is necessary to take the treatment
regularly. Each time you do, you reinforce
the beneficial colonies of bacteria in your
body.

CONSIDER SUPPORTING YOUR DIGESTION WITH SUPPLEMENTS

There are other enzymes, fibers, herbs,
and natural substances for the support of the
digestive process that can be taken in supplement form. Among them are *lactobacillus
sporogenes,* a beneficial intestinal organism
that has proven to reduce populations of
harmful organisms. Also, *fructo-oligosacchar-*

ides (FOS) are naturally occurring carbohydrates that cannot be digested or absorbed by humans but can support the growth of beneficial bacteria. FOS are found in foods like bananas, barley, garlic, honey, onions, wheat, and tomatoes. However, nutritional supplements containing FOS provide a more concentrated source of this compound.

Larch arabinogalactan is an excellent source of dietary fiber that enhances beneficial gut flora and appears to act as an adaptogenic agent on the immune system, lifting up weak aspects and balancing down over-achieving aspects. A chief source of this polysaccharide powder is the wood of the western larch or western tamarack trees. Once an underutilized leftover from the logging industry, larch arabinogalactan has become a valuable supplement.[2]

I've already mentioned other supplementary nutrients that I recommend, such as a hawthorn berry extract, gingerroot powder, bromelain and papain (the enzymes from pineapple and papaya), and fibers like glucomannan and oat bran. Other fibers you can add are arabinogalactan, apple pectin, date fiber powder, and prune powder. The basic digestive enzymes—amylase, cellulase, lactase, lipase, and the proteases—are also available in supplement form. You can find all these items in most good vitamin and health-food centers.

Because all these substances offer definite benefits to a healthy GI tract and promote proper digestion, I have worked with a respected manufacturer of dietary supplements to formulate a product that includes the optimum daily dosages of nineteen herbs, fibers, and enzymes—all in just two capsules a day. It's called Pathway to Healing Digestion Support.

This modestly priced supplement is available directly from the manufacturer, Natural Alternatives, by calling (800) 339–5952, or through the company's Web site: *www.AbundantNutrition.com.*

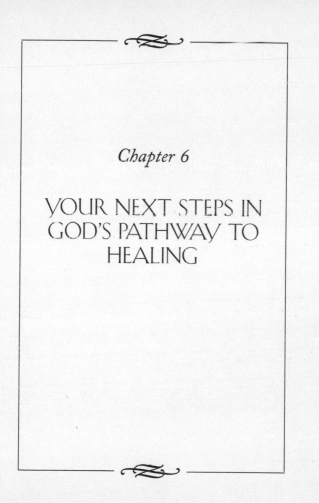

Chapter 6

YOUR NEXT STEPS IN GOD'S PATHWAY TO HEALING

Chapter 6

YOUR NEXT STEPS IN GOD'S PATHWAY TO HEALING

You have begun an important journey toward finding your pathway to healing for digestive problems. Act on the truths you have received.

We want to review and summarize for you the steps you need to take now as you receive God's unique pathway to healing for you.

Step 1: Consult with a physician. Consultation with a physician or a competent medical professional can give you information about your body and give you particular insight as to how to pray for your symptoms. Even better is a Christian physician who will pray the prayer of agreement with you and give you all the facts known about your symptoms of digestive problems.

Step 2: Pray with understanding. Seek God in prayer and ask Him to reveal to you and to your doctor the best steps in the natural that you can take in your pathway to healing.

Step 3: Ask the Holy Spirit to guide you to truth. For some conditions, your doctor may advise you to have surgery or may prescribe particular medications—which sometimes are necessary. God has led us to provide information for our patients about eating a healthy diet, exercising, and taking supplements to provide the enzymes and fiber their body needs. Doing these simple things is very effective in improving your digestion. By referring to the information in this book, you can bring up the discussion of certain natural plant-derived therapies that have been shown to help with digestive problems. Approach your physician by asking if he or she would be willing to work with you to try the natural approach or the prescription approach in combination with the therapies we have discussed. I strongly encourage you to explore all the aspects of the pathway that we have shared with you—the pathway that God has created to strengthen and guard your body. Allow the Holy Spirit to guide you to all truth.

Step 4: Maintain proper and healthy nutrition. Exercise and stay fit. We encourage you to adopt as many principles of a healthy diet as possible and to incorporate into your daily diet the foods, herbs, and natural supplements we have discussed in this book to help your body overcome the symptoms you are battling.

Step 5: Stand firm in God's pathway to healing for you. Refuse to be discouraged or defeated. Be aggressive in prayer and in faith, claiming your healing in Jesus Christ.

We are praying that God will both reveal His pathway to healing for digestive problems to you and give you the strength and faith to walk in it.

ENDNOTES

Chapter 2

1 "All About Enzymes," *MotherNature.com*
   http://www.mothernature.com/articles/
   enzymes/article1 stm

Chapter 3

1. Fiber, Healthwell. *http://www.healthwell.com/*
   healthnotes/Supp/Fiber.cfm.
2. Summarized from Denis P. Burkitt and Peter
   A. James, *The Lancet* (21 July 1973).
3 Herbs and Supplements: Glucomannan, The
   Natural Pharmacist *TNP.com.*

Chapter 4

1. "How Does Your Digestive System Work,"
   Crohns & Colitis Foundation of America,

CCFA Weekly Features. *http://www.ccfa.org*

2. Digestive Organs, Texas Virtual Clinic—Digestive Organs. *http://websurg.ith.tmc.edu/digestive/organs.html.*

3. Michael Schachter, M.D., F.A.C.A.M., "Introduction to the Digestive System," HealthWorld Online—Integrative Medicine. *http://www.healthy.net.*

Chapter 5

1. Acidophilus (Probiotics) and Fructo-Oligo-saccharides (FOS), *MotherNature.com*, Health Encyclopedia.

2. Anonymous, Larch arabinogalactan. *Alternative Medicine Review.* (Oct. 2000): 5: 463–66.

REGINALD B. CHERRY, M.D.—A MEDICAL DOCTOR'S TESTIMONY

The first six years of my life were lived in the dusty rural town of Mansfield, in the Ouachita Mountains of western Arkansas. In those childhood years, I had one seemingly impossible dream—to become a doctor!

Through God's grace, I attended and graduated from Baylor University and the University of Texas Medical School. Throughout those years, I felt God tug on my heart a number of times, especially through Billy Graham, as I heard him preach on television. But I never surrendered my life to Jesus Christ.

In those early days of practicing medicine, I met Dr. Kenneth Cooper and became trained in the field of preventive medicine. In the midseventies I moved to Houston and established a medical practice for preventive medicine. Sadly, at that time money became a driving force in my life.

Nevertheless, God was so good to me. He brought into our clinic a nurse who became a Spirit-filled Christian, and she began praying for me. In fact, she had her whole church praying for me!

In my search for fulfillment and meaning in life, I called out to God one night in late November of 1979 and prayed, "Jesus, I give you everything I own. I'm sorry for the life I've lived. I want to live for you the rest of my days. I give you my life." A doctor had been born again. Oh, and by the way, that beautiful nurse who had prayed for me and shared Jesus with me is Linda, who is now my wife!

Not only did Jesus transform my life, but He also transformed my medical practice. God spoke to me and said, "I want you to establish a Christian clinic. From now on when you practice medicine, you will be *ministering* to patients." I began to pray for patients, seeking God's pathway to healing in the supernatural realm as well as in the natural realm.

Over the years we have witnessed how

God has miraculously used both supernatural and natural pathways to heal our patients and to demonstrate His marvelous healing and saving power.

I know what God has done in my life, and I know what God has done in the lives of our patients. He can do the same in yours—He has a unique pathway to healing for you! He is the Lord that heals you (see Exodus 15:26), and by His stripes you were healed (see Isaiah 53:5).

Know that Linda and I are standing with you as you seek God's pathway to healing for digestive problems, and as you walk in His pathway to healing for your life.

If you do not know Jesus Christ as your personal Lord and Savior, I invite you to pray this prayer and ask Jesus into your life:

Lord Jesus, I invite you into my life as my Lord and Savior. I repent of my past sins. I ask you to forgive me. Thank you for shedding your blood on the cross to cleanse me from my sin and to heal me. I receive your gift of everlasting life and surrender all to you. Thank you, Jesus, for saving me. Amen.

ABOUT THE AUTHOR

Reginald B. Cherry, M.D., did his pre-med at Baylor University, graduated from the University of Texas Medical School, and has practiced diagnostic and preventive medicine for more than twenty-five years. His work in medicine has been recognized and honored by the city of Houston and President George W. Bush when he was the governor of Texas.

Dr. Cherry and his wife, Linda, a clinical nurse who has worked with Dr. Cherry and his patients during the past two-and-a-half decades, now host the popular television program *The Doctor and the Word*, which has a potential viewing audience of 90 million homes weekly. They also publish a monthly medical newsletter and produce topical audiocassette teachings, minibooks, and booklets. Dr. Cherry is author of the bestselling books *The Doctor and the Word*, *The Bible Cure*, and *Healing Prayer*.

RESOURCES AVAILABLE FROM REGINALD B. CHERRY MINISTRIES, INC.

Prayers That Heal: Faith-Building Prayers When You Need a Miracle

Combining the wisdom of over twenty-five years of medical practice and the revelation of God's Word, Dr. Cherry provides the knowledge you need to pray effectively against diabetes, cancer, heart disease, eye problems, hypoglycemia, and fifteen other common afflictions that try to rob you of your health.

Healing Prayer

A fascinating in-depth look at a vital link between spiritual and physical healing. Dr. Cherry presents actual case histories of people healed through prayer, plus the latest information on herbs, vitamins, and supplements that promote vibrant health. This is sound information you need to keep you healthy—mind, soul, and body.

God's Pathway to Healing: Prostate Cancer

This minibook is packed with enlightening insights for men who are searching for ways to prevent prostate cancer or who have actually been diagnosed with this disease. Discover how foods, plant-derived natural supplements, and a change in diet can be incorporated into your life to help you find a pathway to healing for prostate disease.

God's Pathway to Healing: Herbs That Heal

Learn the truth about common herbal remedies and discover the possible side effects of each.

Discover which herbs can help treat symptoms of insomnia, arthritis, heart problems, asthma, and many other conditions. Read this book and see if herbs are part of God's pathway to healing for you.

God's Pathway to Healing: Menopause

This minibook is full of helpful advice for women who are going through what can be a very stressful time of life. Find out what foods, supplements, and steps can be taken to find a pathway to healing for menopause and perimenopause.

The Bible Cure (now in paperback)

Dr. Cherry presents hidden truths in the Bible taken from ancient dietary health laws, how Jesus anointed with natural substances to heal, and how to activate faith through prayer for health and healing. This book validates scientific medical research by proving God's original health plan.

The Doctor and the Word (now in paperback)

Dr. Cherry introduces how God has a pathway to healing for you. Jesus healed instantaneously and supernaturally, while other healings involved a process. Discover how the manifestation of your healing can come about by seeking His ways.

Dr. Cherry's *Study Guides, Volume 2* (bound volume)

Receive thirty valuable resource study guides from topics Dr. Cherry has taught on the Trinity Broadcasting Network (TBN) program *The Doctor and the Word*.

Basic Nutrient Support

Dr. Cherry has developed a daily nutrient supplement that is the simplest to take and yet the most complete supplement available today. Protect your body daily with natural substances that fight cancer, heart disease, and many other problems.

Call Natural Alternatives at (800) 339–5952 to place your order. Mention service code "BN30" when ordering. (Or order through the company's Web site: *www.AbundantNutrition.com.*)

Digestion Support

You don't have to struggle with the painful and embarrassing effects of poor digestion. Dr. Cherry has formulated a potent supplement containing the key nutrients and extracts from natural substances. Based on his twenty-five years of medical practice and research, this supplement includes everything he recommends to support digestive health. Call Natural Alternatives at (800) 339–5952 to place your order. Mention service code "K263" when ordering. (Or order through the company's Web site: *www.Abundant Nutrition.com.*)

Reginald B. Cherry Ministries, Inc.
P.O. Box 27711
Houston, TX 77227-7711
1-888-DRCHERRY

BECOME A PATHWAY TO HEALING PARTNER

We invite you to become a "pathway partner." We ask you to stand with us in prayer and financial support as we provide new programs, resources, books, mini-books, and a one-of-a-kind monthly newsletter.

Our monthly *Pathway to Healing Partner Newsletter* sorts through the confusion about health and healing. In it, Dr. Cherry shares sensible, biblical, and medical steps you can take to get well. Every issue points you to your pathway to healing. Writing from a Christian physician's Bible-based point of view, Dr. Cherry talks about nutrition and health, how to pray for specific diseases, updates on the latest medical research, Linda's own recipes for healthy eating, and questions and answers about issues you need to know about.

In addition, we'll provide you with Dr. Cherry and Linda's ministry calendar, broadcast schedule, resources for better living, and special monthly offers.

This newsletter is available to you as you partner with the Cherrys through prayer and monthly financial support to help expand this God-given ministry. Pray today about responding with a monthly contribution of $10 or more. Call or write to the following address to find out how you can receive this valuable information.

Become a pathway partner today by writing:

> Reginald B. Cherry Ministries, Inc.
> P.O. Box 27711
> Houston, TX 77227-7711

Visit our Web site:
www.drcherry.org

1-888-DRCHERRY